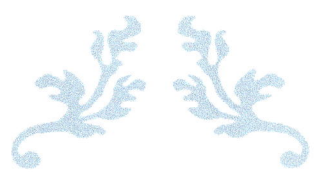

KAMA SUTRA FOR BEGINNERS

A Complete Beginners Guide To Boost Your Couple's
Pleasure And Improve Intimacy In Your Relationship.
Tantric Sex And Sex Positions For Men And Woman

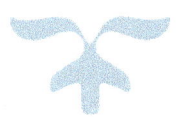

Melany Evans

Kama Sutra for Beginners

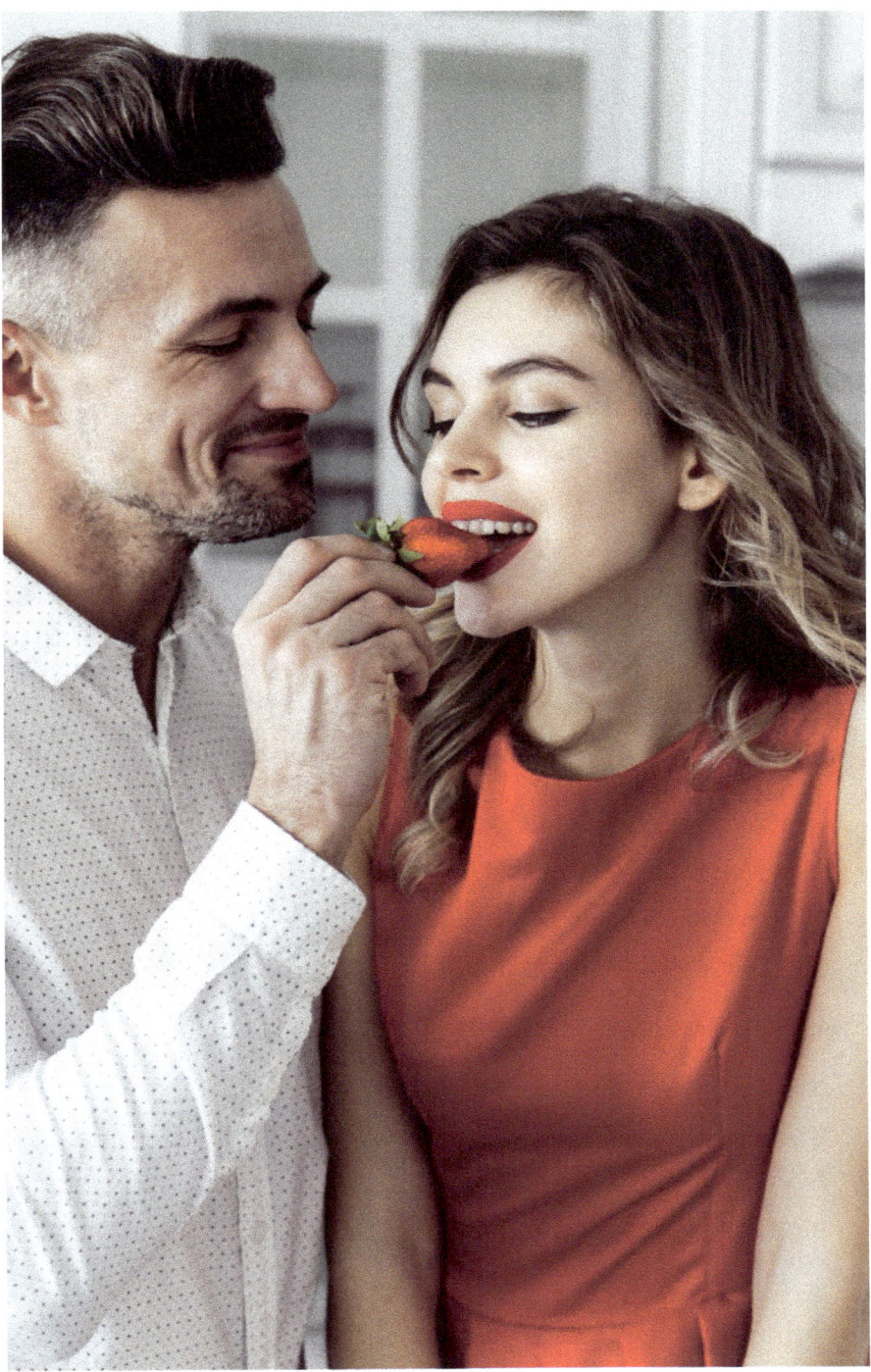

Table of Contents

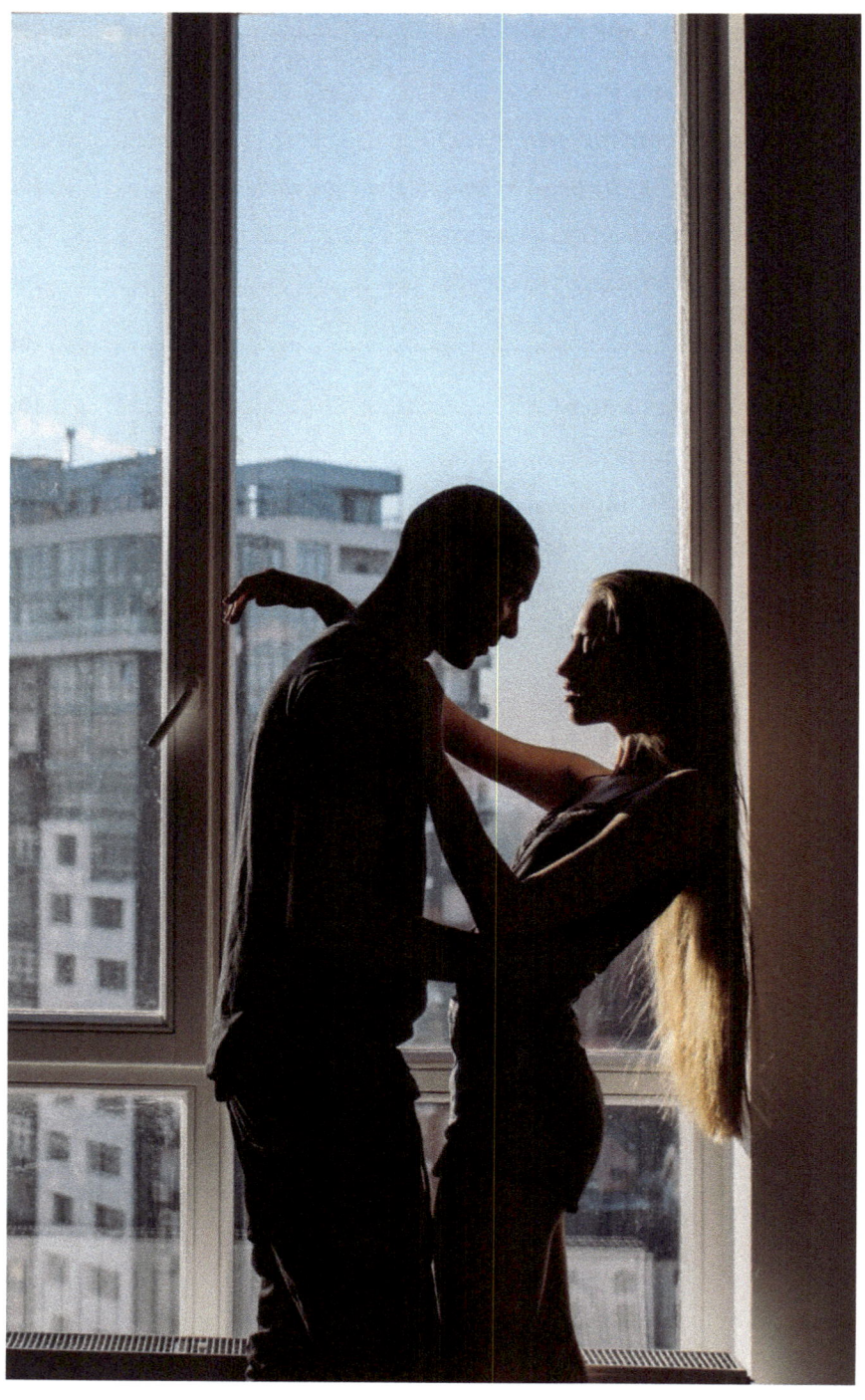

INTRODUCTION

T antric sex is tied in with regarding one's body and the body of one's accomplice. By setting aside some effort to become acquainted with one's own body just as that of one's accomplice, it can help make the experience satisfying for the two individuals.

An individual may consider giving their accomplice a moderate, full-body back rub to find out about their body and help stir their sexual energy. This may likewise enable an individual to become in line with their accomplice's needs and wants.

Similar to the case with any sexual activity, if anytime an individual or their accomplice gets awkward, the movement should stop.

There are a couple of things an individual or couple can never really plan for tantric sex. For instance, they can:

- **Put aside time**: Tantric sex is tied in with moving gradually and being at the time. Sometimes, it can be most recent an hour or more. Therefore, make certain to put aside some an ideal opportunity to completely connect with and appreciate the experience.

- **Set up the brain**: Focusing on the second can be difficult if an individual is encountering pressure or has numerous things at the forefront of their thoughts. Contemplating or extending before tantric sex may help accomplish an unmistakable attitude.

- **Locate a decent spot**: Environment has a critical part in tantric sex. In a perfect world, it will happen in a loosening upsetting with an agreeable temperature. An individual might need to diminish the lights, light a scented flame, or put on loosening up music. To construct the second with oneself, an individual can attempt the accompanying tips:

- **Practice care:** Tantric sex urges individuals to be available at the time. An individual should zero in on their breathing and substantial sensations.

11

- **Investigate the body**: Giving a self-knead in which the individual focuses on their touch and body may help uplift actual sensations and excitement.

- **Stroke off**: An individual may wish to take part in tantric confidence. Like with cooperated sex, the objective of this may not be the climax. All things considered, individuals may do this to attempt to feel more associated with their own bodies.

Tantric Sex sounds strange and something that solitary eastern spiritualists may know anything about. In fact, the act of tantric sex uncovers to us the key to recover our sexual closeness and revive the lost enthusiasm. Learning the privileged insights of tantric sex and new couples having intercourse positions will guarantee that you will encounter new delights into the sensual and extend your sexual information. To fabricate the second with an accomplice, individuals can attempt the accompanying tips:

- **Receive a hand-on-heart position**: To increase a profound association, couples ought to sit with folded legs and face one another. The two accomplices should put their correct hand on the other's heart, with the left hand on their partner's. Feel the association and attempt to synchronize relaxing.

- **Try not to go direct**: Normally, sexual exercises may follow a content of foreplay, intercourse, and climax. Nonetheless, tantric sex is tied in with testing, so it is ideal to remain open to what particularly feels great at the time.

- **Visually connect**: Making eye to eye connection may help extend the association and increase closeness.

- **Take things moderate**: Tantric sex is reflective and about investigating sensations at the time. This cycle should be a moderate and agreeable excursion for the two accomplices.

Breathing is a necessary piece of tantric sex. This is halfway because tantric sex rotates around contemplation.

During tantric sex, an individual should zero in on breathing profoundly through the stomach. To accomplish this, they should take a full breath through the nose for five tallies. They should feel their stomach expand. They should then breathe out through the mouth for five checks.

When participating in tantric sex with an accomplice, synchronizing the breath may build association and closeness.

Another breathing procedure individuals can attempt is Kapalbhati. Kapalbhati drags out discharge in guys. When a male feels that they are going to discharge, they ought to strongly breathe out through the mouth, then take part in a programmed breathe in through the mouth.

Except if you're dating a mystic, your accomplice can't guess what you might be thinking. When you vocalize what feels better, what needs some work, or that your clitoris is only somewhat higher, and you'd truly love it if your accomplice could concentrate all their vitality there, then you both advantage.

When you can both say what you like and how you like it, you're not very far away from saying how it affects you. From that point, the dirty talk will simply stream — it will take practice, obviously.

Along these lines, perhaps your rendition of talking dirty right presently is telling your accomplice that you're going to come. That is generally one part of dirty talk that individuals can handle, yet simply consider how hot it would be to simply let free and uncover all the things you keep in your mind during sex.

Before you know it, you've gone from hollering, "I'm coming! I'm coming!" to something about how you're going to appear at your accomplice's work, lock them in their office, and give them the sort of mid-day break that you've both constantly needed. At that time you've made a dream and a situation that you can hold returning to and can expand upon. Perhaps you'll even wind up receiving your own adaptation of Fifty Shades of Gray in return — you never know!

As any specialist or sex advisor will let you know, foreplay is a critical piece of sex, particularly for ladies. It takes ladies far longer to get stirred than men, and that is the reason they don't climax as fast as men do. For us, foreplay is basic.

If you can begin with some dirty talk, then you'll be enticing each other in manners that are similarly as significant as physical foreplay. Quick ones are fun, yet if you have the opportunity to take as much time as is needed, then do it. Put aside an entire 20 minutes of simply talking dirty to one another before you even take off your garments and contact one another. You'll see the difference it makes.

It's constantly pleasant when you can even now astound yourself, right? Furthermore, the thing is, when you drive yourself to accomplish something that you've never done, you very well might understand it was made for you. Talking graphically about how you need to be touched and how you're going to touch your accomplice may upset your sexual coexistence — however you find out, unless you check it out.

There are a lot of approaches to zest things up in your long haul relationship when things are feeling somewhat stale. If your sexual coexistence has become the stuff of evangelist directly before bed, then talking dirty to your accomplice is a simple method to change it up a piece.

Odds are the dirty things you've been thinking, yet haven't said so anyone can hear yet, will really amaze them. You can murmur in your accomplice's ear, ensuring your lips just marginally brush their ear cartilage. From that point, contingent upon their reaction, you can proceed or let them dominate and mention to you what they're thinking,

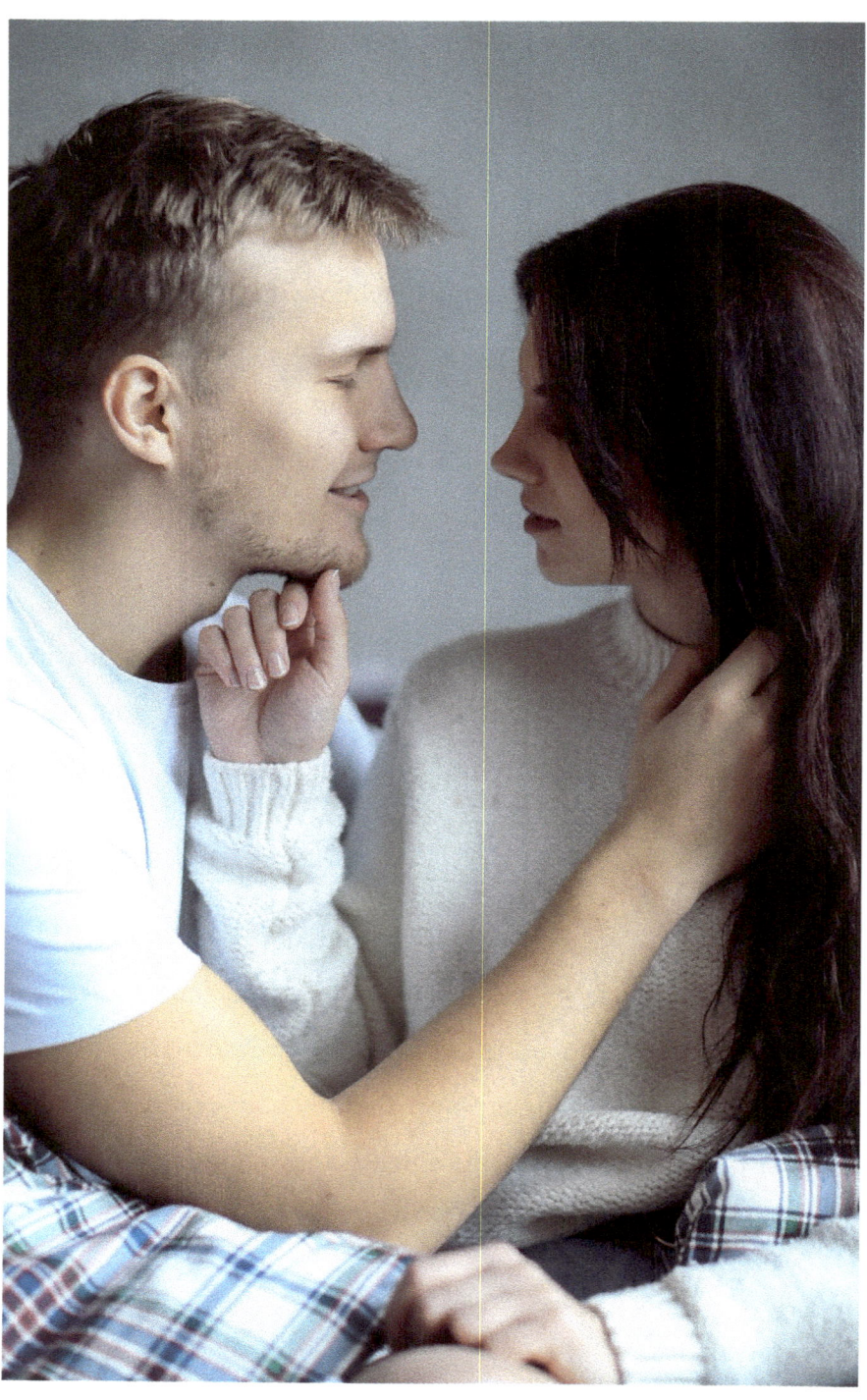

CHAPTER 1. SLOWING DOWN IN SEX

While enthusiastic and furious sex meetings are great, more slow, exotic experiences infrequently get a similar consideration. What's more, they should! Hindering sex is probably the best thing you can accomplish for your pleasure.

Great Vibrations sexologist Carol Queen, Ph.D., clarifies: "More slow sex and a more extended development can bring about more grounded climaxes for some individuals (a basic correlation is that you're developing a 'charge' in your body that discharges with peak, and a more drawn out charge can inspire a more grounded reaction)."

There are things you can do even before you get into the room that can assist you with easing back things down. For one, practice care, recommends August McLaughlin, creator of Girl Boner.

Download a contemplation application to use before bed or first thing when you awaken, and you'll before long figure out how to be more careful and present in all circumstances. "Anything that encourages check out our bodies and wants and deliveries stress can make sex all the more engaging and pleasurable," she adds.

This substance is imported from {embed-name}. You might have the option to locate a similar substance in another arrangement, or you might have the option to discover more data at their site.

And keeping in mind that planning time between the sheets may appear to be nonsensical to sexiness, it can really help facilitate your psyche and give you, to a lesser extent, a period smash to rush to the end goal.

Sex and relationship master Mackenzie Riel, of TooTimid.com, clarifies, "Sex can get hurried when there's not sufficient opportunity to get to the development that happens just before the peak." Without stressing over rising promptly the following day or some other obligations, you'd be amazed how much more liberated you are to appreciate each other's bodies. "[Scheduling sex] may feel senseless, however when you have the opportunity to truly appreciate each other without stress or obligation, you have more opportunity to construct the sexual strain." says Riel.

"When you have the opportunity to truly appreciate each other without stress or obligation, you have more opportunity to manufacture sexual pressure."

You may likewise need to give edging (or climax control) an attempt. Consider it like stretch preparing for competitors, says McLaughlin. By getting exceptionally near climax and afterward halting just previously, you'll get increasingly more stimulated each time.

When you at the last climax, it'll feel substantially more extreme than ordinary climaxes. Notwithstanding, McLaughlin notes, you ought to examine edging previously with your accomplice, so you're both mindful of the objective in the long game.

This can even be essential for the fun, as you're prodding each other to the edge of climax just to ease off.

This substance is imported from {embed-name}. You might have the option to locate a similar substance in another arrangement, or you might have the option to discover more data at their site.

When the garments do fall off, there are a couple of things to remember. "This sort of sex is more profound than interfacing actually," says New York City sex advisor Joy Davidson, Ph.D., creator of Fearless Sex. "It's tied in with losing yourself at the time and holding sincerely as well."

This sort of licentious association isn't about insta-climax. "It's tied in with appreciating each touch and sensation, which magnifies the physical and passionate experience," says sexologist Trina Read, DHS, from Calgary, Canada. It additionally brings about a greater result when you do hit the large O. "The sexual strain of expectation prompts a more serious peak," says Laura Berman, Ph.D., creator of The Passion Prescription: 10 Weeks to Your Best Sex Ever.

To shield yourselves from running to the end goal, lie in bed simply kissing and touching. "This common incitement places you in a reflective state, permitting you to focus in on every sensation," says Davidson. Treat him to an enticing encounter by contacting him from head to toe. "Getting comfortable with the subtleties of his life structures lets you work on a higher sexy level," says Berman.

So let your hands skim down his spine. Run your fingers along the wrinkle where his thigh meets his crotch.

Then let him explore your randy locales as well. "Revealing delight guides specific toward your bodies resemble a mystery you two offer," says Davidson. "It's another selective feature of your relationship."

The Most Effective Method to Have Hella Romantic Sex

It might seem as though a great deal of hot air, however, taking as one can cause you both to feel completely associated.

"When you are so centered around getting into a similar beat, you enter a close to trancelike state," says Read. "It brings you into the 'zone,' where you're profoundly mindful of your person, and your outer climate appears to blur to dark."

To synchronize your breathing, get into a body-to-body position, for example, spooning or coital arrangement. Or then again, sit nose-to-nose with your legs folded over one another and your hands on one another's chests so you can feel your pulses.

Then breathe in and breathe out, gradually and purposely, giving uncommon consideration to your man's movement as you stroke and kiss. "Taking couple helps your energy levels ascend at a similar rate as well," says Read. "It causes you to feel actually merged."

"It causes you to feel genuinely merged."

Perhaps the most ideal approach to enjoy an extraordinary suggestive experience—and appreciate each tasty second—is to keep yourself from seeing and hearing diverting sensations.

"Cutting off sight and sound intensifies sex in two different ways," says Berman. "Killing all potential aggravations keeps you fixated on the second and one another. Additionally, erasing one sense permits the others to turn out to be more intense, so you can truly check out the delight you're giving one another. You make a sweeping exotic trade."

Sentimental Sex Positions

To get into lewd focus mode, dump the temperament music and sentimental lighting. You need complete quietness and obscurity. (This would be an ideal chance to draw out those blindfolds.) As you stroke your man, truly home in on how he feels and tastes and scents. Make an effort not to make a peep... except for the groans and moans that thoughtlessly get away from your lips. Figure out the surface of his skin, tune in to his beating heart as his excitement raises, and nestle him all finished so you can breathe in his pith. Simultaneously, permit yourself to get lost in all that he's doing to you. "Try not to feel like you have to perform for him or be as boisterous as a pornography star," says Berman. "Simply unwind and revel in the stunning joy he's giving you."

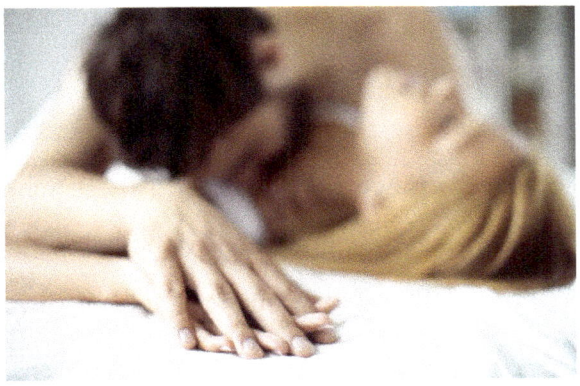

Step-by-Step Instructions to Give Your Guy a Tantric Massage

While shutting out interruptions lets you center internally and zoom in around your sensations, looking at your accomplice constrains you to focus on one another.

"Numerous ladies feel secluded during sex because you both will in general turn out to be so up to speed in your own actual joy, you dismiss the other individual," clarifies Berman. "In any case, visually connecting is an approach to impart. It overcomes that issue and lets you truly know about your man's quality."

This doesn't imply that you ought to get into a gazing challenge with your person. It's more similar to you're peering inside him as opposed to exactly at him. Study his outward appearance and attempt to envision his opinion and feeling, particularly when he approaches climax. "There's something so soul-uncovering about observing your accomplice right then and there when he's open and helpless," says Read. "Bolting each other's look at this closest to home second is somewhat similar to stating to one another 'I confide in you.' You have to feel really reinforced with somebody to share that sort of acknowledgment."

It takes ladies a normal of 13 minutes longer than men to have a climax. That is a serious hop.

I don't think about you, however, getting off quickly is just conceivable when only I'm with my Hitachi Magic Wand. "The climax hole is incorporated with our different male and female physiology," says Wendy Strgar, loveologist, and originator of the grease organization Good Clean Love.

We must locate a functional answer to this issue. Everybody has the right to have a climax during sex. It's an implicit understanding of intercourse: You get to climax, I get to climax, and everybody is cheerful.

Anyway, what do we do? We must back sex off.

Presently, I'm supportive of that firm fast in and out, don't misunderstand me, yet if mom will come, we need to decelerate speed to build the chance of climax, shutting the hole for the last time.

God favors America.

Sex Starts the Moment We Enter the Space

Sex doesn't begin the moment we get the P in the V. It starts the second we choose to get lively: from foreplay to sexual contacting, to all out intercourse.

"Hindering the time, giving ourselves more opportunity to be interested and investigate joy, helps the two sexes," Strgar says. "Removing the center [to] surge toward intercourse facilitates the tension about the sexual exhibition. Entrance ought to consistently follow [a] clitoral climax because the female blossom[s] with this sort of delight."

This implies ensuring you appropriately set up your S.O's. woman blossom prior to going to the max.

Foreplay the Entire Day

To back sex off, you must back foreplay off. For a significant number of us anxious monstrosities (myself included), foreplay can get ignored seemingly out of the blue.

One second you're kissing, the following second you have an entrance. It's OK - it happens to potentially anyone.

"Multiplying your [foreplay] time will change the peak, however the relationship itself," Strgar says. "Give those additional minutes to [a] erotic back rub." You can likewise attempt a little light quill play with a tickler or some areola incitement. Remember the intensity of touch! Run your hands everywhere on your accomplice's body with delicate tickles, scouring, even light scratching. Postponing the headliner will manufacture expectation... also, excitement.

"Observe how it feels to simply rub the sanctuaries, the inward thighs, the sacrum," Strgar says. "Sexual joy spots exist everywhere on the body, and every one elevates genital reaction."

Think Carefully

Strgar says having great sex is tied in with having the option to quiet your mind and be at the time. "Divert your outlook about sex from execution (or accomplishment) to detecting and growing joy in the entirety of its structures."

The cerebrum is the most grounded sex organ we have. The capacity to fantasize and center our cerebrums to open our bodies to delight can be the difference between climax and disappointment.

Keep in mind, it's not about how you perform during sex - it's tied in with appreciating the experience.

Improve Your Faculties

Another approach to upgrade foreplay is to zero in on the entirety of your faculties, not simply contact.

Strgar encourages focusing on your accomplice's taste. It will keep you at the time, and more drew in, the two of which make experiences limitlessly more sexual. Tune in to the sounds being made, which are additionally exceptionally educational while you joy one another.

Aroma is another huge one in the room. Fundamental oils work like aphrodisiacs: Put a little jasmine on your inward wrist to get your accomplice in the state of mind. Trust me on this.

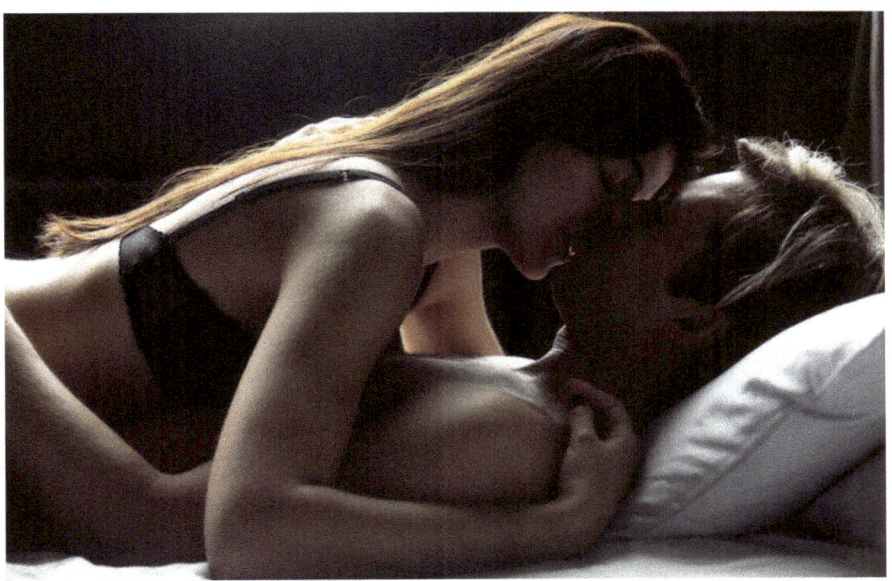

Lastly, Sex

Truly, the sex itself is likewise significant, individuals. When you've truly upgraded practically each and every sensitive spot known to man, you'll presumably be reeling to get that penetrative circumstance moving.

One moment! In any event, during intercourse, you should be at the time. Strgar says' everything regarding the strokes - you need to fluctuate between full-profundity peen and exceptional, shallow jumps.

"Hinder entrance by utilizing different sorts of strokes, making designs that the two accomplices are following [both shallow and deep]," she says. "Space the profound ones as far separated as you can, for as long as could be expected under the circumstances."

This sort of affection making isn't only extraordinary for delight, yet in addition, your relationship overall. "It will astonish you and furthermore unite you during intercourse," Strgar says. What's more, that, obviously, is useful for everybody - and their climaxes.

As indicated by late examination, American heterosexual sex endures just 7.3 minutes by and large. What's the surge, individuals? If we contrast sex with eating, Americans are what might be compared to a cheap food joint-an In-N-Out, if you will.

Sex, similar to food, should be enjoyed. It should be a four-course supper.

You don't simply stroll into an extravagant café and request your primary course. You take as much time as is needed. For what reason is that solitary 29% of ladies report continually arriving at a climax during sex contrasted with that of 75% of men?

This could have to do with the term of sex. It bodes well that fewer ladies report arriving at climax if it takes somebody with a vulva 10 to 20 minutes to arrive at climax, all things considered, versus that of a somebody with a penis (For individuals with penises, the normal time between first infiltration and climax is two and three minutes.)

The Benefits of Slow Sex

If you think about the normal length of sex and the differences in our particular climax times, somebody is plainly getting the great part of the bargain here, and it isn't the individuals who have a vagina.

This could be clarified by the overall absence of instruction with respect to the clitoris in the United States, or it very well may be because of the male-driven thoughts of sexual joy that ruled our way of life, yet hindering sex could be the response to a considerable lot of our socio-social sex aberrations.

We at Good Clean Love have faith in equivalent joy, the idea that sex ought to be similarly fulfilling for all people included. For this situation, equivalent joy implies taking as much time as necessary. Furthermore, prepare to have your mind blown.

Hindering your sex life: being cozier, lengthening foreplay, differing your sexual positions, playing with toys and lube… it upgrades the experience for everybody included!

Equity among people is helpful for more sure, satisfying, and practical relationships. In pretty much every examination, the two people report wishing their sex kept going longer.

In spite of hurtful marks of disgrace, ladies can appreciate sex the same amount as men, and men want sentimental consideration similarly as much as ladies.

Slow sex, as moderate food, could be a piece of the development towards a more drawn out enduring, more economical, comprehensive way to deal with carrying on with life.

Considering sex a greater amount of an encounter and less of a demonstration is pivotal in grasping sexiness and sexuality. So how about we take a little exercise from the turtle and the bunny and transform this cheap food sex into a top-notch food experience.

Keen on hindering your more cozy minutes? We've arranged an elite of six stunts to help get you there.

1. Play with Scents

For what reason accomplishes it work? Aromas animate the limbic cerebrum, which is related to memory, sexuality, and feeling. The limbic framework seems, by all accounts, to be fundamentally liable for our passionate life, and has a ton to do with the arrangement of recollections.

Easing back things somewhere near zeroing in on aromas previously and during sex could trigger excitement and make the experience more paramount for you and your accomplice.

Despite the fact that, be careful of what fragrances you are picking. In excess of 95 percent of the synthetic compounds in engineered scents are gotten from petrochemicals. Stay away from artificial aromas and search for every single common decision.

2. Use Lube in Unexpected Ways

Examination with elective uses for lube by placing it in surprising spots. For instance, look to the regular bends of your accomplice's body – their neck, their lower back, hips, or inward thighs. These additional couple of moments of play will lengthen the term of sex and improve the experience.

3. Act Shy

There's not at all like adding a little anticipation to elevate the experience and moderate things down.

The exemplary round of acting shy and making your accomplice sit tight for their peak is another stunt to have moderate sex. The act of "edging," or "climax preparing" adds more opportunity to your foreplay and lengthens the time paving the way to climax, prompting a more elevated encounter for you and your accomplice.

3. Visually Connect

Joining eye to eye connection to your sex is another simple stunt to have moderate sex. Eye to eye connection is an offer of regard, comprehension, and interest.

Taking a gander at someone else is a method of getting input on specific focuses. It is likewise utilized as a synchronizing signal. Take a few minutes to bolt eyes and hold the eye to eye connection for sexier commitment.

Not exclusively will this add some an ideal opportunity to your daily schedule, you can interface with your accomplice in a more important manner.

4. Invest More Energy on Kissing

Have you ever known about a philematologist? All things considered, they are researchers who study kissing, and they have discovered some pretty cool science to back why everybody ought to invest more energy making out.

Kissing can lessen pulse, consumes calories, and builds levels of your "vibe great" synthetic substances serotonin, dopamine, and oxytocin in your cerebrum. Look at this article, 8 medical advantages of kissing, to find out additional.

Stir up your typical daily schedule by investing more energy making out during sex. Discover fun approaches to upgrade your kisses, for instance, utilizing all common love oils all the rage on the body.

5. Zero in on Your Breathing

Another tip on the best way to have moderate sex is dominating breathing strategies in the room. This can be critical to lengthening the term of your sex because it can assist you with enduring longer.

Taking full breaths can improve your odds of having moderate sex because it builds oxygen levels in the blood, which advances unwinding all through the body.

Work on taking some full breaths whenever you become involved with the second to pull together your energy to maintain a strategic distance from untimely discharge.

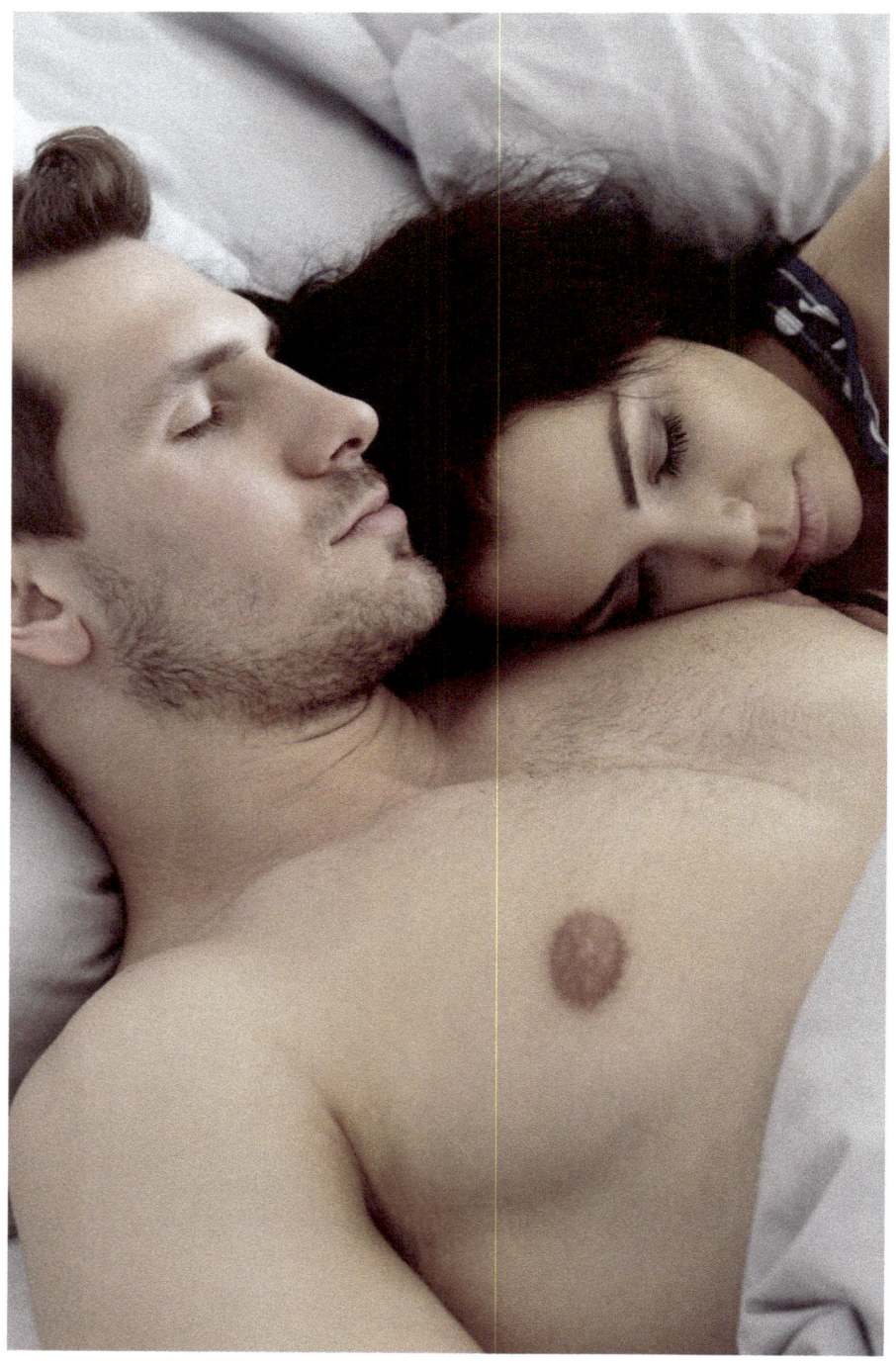

CHAPTER 2. MALE AND FEMALE EROGENOUS ZONE

Yet, there are really numerous different zones of the body that can be associated with sex and foreplay outside of those couple of key spots. Ever have that very scrumptious shivery inclination when your accomplice kowtows and down your neck? That is because the neck is what's called an erogenous zone. If you're searching for additional approaches to zest things up in the room, investigate our guide for all the undiscovered delight zones you've been passing up.

"Erogenous Zone": Where Have I Heard That Before?

If you're a sitcom watcher, you may have heard the expression "erogenous zone" previously. Recall that scene of Friends when Monica clarifies the seven female erogenous zones to Chandler?

Who could fail to remember the sublime "SEVEN, SEVEN, SEVEN!"- gasm she polishes off with?

Another important clasp is scene three in season five of How I Met Your Mother, including a note pad on "Robin 101." Ted's case that scouring Robin's left knee truly does it for her ends up being false, yet the knee really can be an erogenous zone!

Erogenous Zone Definition

If you're considering how the left knee might be sexy, the appropriate response is pretty straightforward. Any portion of the body can really be an erogenous zone.

An erogenous zone is a region of the body with elevated affectability that can create a sexual reaction when animated.

41

Erogenous zones are additional delicate because of centralizations of sensitive spots in these regions.

Erogenous Zones Chart

Since you understand what an erogenous zone is, you might be pondering where you can discover yours.

The Top 10 Female Erogenous Zones

Outside of the standard suspects, here's our rundown for the best erogenous zones for ladies to give a shot alongside tips for invigorating these delicate areas.

From your own encounters, you've presumably found how delicate these regions can be when invigorated by an accomplice.

1. Your Ears

Your ears contain several tactile receptors inside, and the external skin is additionally touchy. Because of this present, it's ideal to be delicate when invigorating the ears.

Have your accomplice gently follow the outside of your ear, and afterward move in to kiss and snack the ear cartilage. You may likewise appreciate murmuring or delicate blowing to get that shivery, goosebumps feeling.

2. The Nape of Your Neck

A great many people center around the throat when things get warmed, yet the scruff or back of the neck is another hot zone. Contingent upon the position, it very well may be difficult for your accomplice to arrive at the scruff of your neck with their lips, however, a light touch with the tip of their fingers can feel astounding.

They can invigorate the touchy sensitive spots with light strokes while kissing, and run their fingernails down the rear of your neck to create a shivery shudder.

3. Your Butt

This one may not be too stunning, however, numerous ladies naturally dismiss the butt if they realize they hate the butt-centric play. Try not to thump it till you attempt it!

There's no compelling reason to avoid the behind because you partner it with all out infiltration. Having your accomplice touch the external skin or, in any event, doing some light fingering is an extraordinary method to exploit the various delicate nerve closes inside your rear-end. A few ladies even appreciate delicate licking!

4. Your Fingertips

Consider it: Your fingertips are one of the most touchy zones of your body. In spite of the fact that we don't, for the most part, consider fingers being sexy, clasping hands or delicately stimulating the fingertips during sex is both sexual and private.

To kick it up a score, your accomplice can gently suck on every one of your fingers, each in turn. Keeping in touch is basic here to completely feel the consideration being showered on you.

5. Your Lower Back

The nerves in the little of your back, or sacrum, are associated with your pelvis, making this area touchy to sexual incitement. Regardless of whether it's the tickle of a light touch or more strong weight, numerous ladies discover this sort of tactile play engaging.

If you need to get inventive with it, take a stab at exploring different avenues regarding temperatures utilizing an ice 3D square or warmth cushion.

… And the Ones You May Have Forgotten

So perhaps those were somewhat self-evident, however, you likely didn't see these coming! Here are a couple of more spots that are certainly worth testing.

6. Your Inner Wrists

This delicate heartbeat point can be an incredible method to kick the activity off. Daintily touch the skin of the inward wrist to get your accomplice moving, and later on, this can advance to kissing and delicate licking.

Part of the allure with this zone is the "threat" factor: your accomplice has assumed responsibility for one of your most weak regions.

7. Your Armpits

Believe it or not, the armpits are an erogenous zone! There's nothing similar to a little stimulation to make the move from senseless to sexy.

Consider how responsive and sensitive your armpit is — this can be converted into sexual affectability. Start with light contacting, and gradually quicken into brisker movements. The sentiment of being tickled yet in addition, stirred can be exciting.

8. Your Scalp

The scalp is crammed with sensitive spots — simply consider how pleasant it feels when somebody plays with your hair. While kissing, your accomplice should run their fingernails through your hair and along your scalp to invigorate that shivery inclination.

Zeroing in on the scruff of the neck or the rear of the ears while doing this can be a too hot approach to animate numerous erogenous zones on the double.

9. Your Stomach

This is a zone that you can exploit without anyone else or with an accomplice. The way into this erogenous zone is prodding. It's so near the peril zone that contacting this zone can really advance the progression of blood to your clit and vagina.

Light, prodding contacts with your accomplice's tongue and fingertips are the most ideal approaches to animate this erogenous zone, alongside temperature play utilizing an ice 3D square or cold washcloth.

10. Your Knees

Much the same as Ted claims about Robin in How I Met Your Mother, having your accomplice animate the rear of your knee can really be too sexy.

Once more, this has to do with the affectability of the district and how sensitive it is. Have your accomplice knead your legs during foreplay, giving extraordinary consideration to the rear of your knee utilizing both their fingers and tongue.

Outside of the typical suspects, here's our rundown for the best erogenous zones for ladies to give a shot alongside tips for animating these touchy districts.

Step by Step Instructions to Know Which Erogenous Zone You'll Like

The best way to truly sort out which of your erogenous zones are most touchy is to give them a shot. Affectability shifts from individual to individual, and there is certainly not a specific method to tell which spots will be the best turn-ons for you. If you sense that you're stuck between a rock and a hard place, don't worry! We've picked a couple of zones you can begin to try different things with dependent on your character and most successive beverage request.

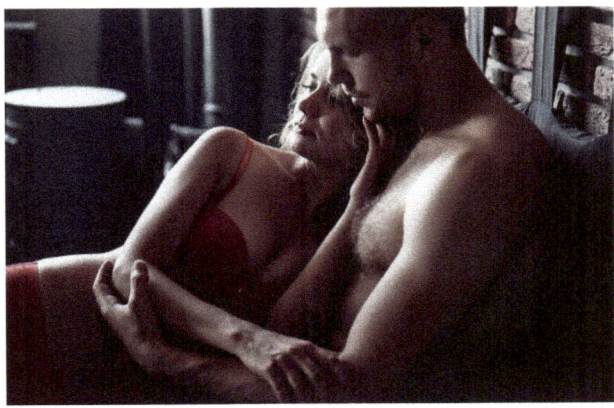

Ladies' Erogenous Zones versus Men's Erogenous Zones

Despite the fact that we're principally centered around the women for this guide, it very well may be a decent beginning stage for men as well. Outside of the privates, ladies and men really share similar erogenous zones. Similarly as ladies may discover joy outside the clit and vagina, men can, in all honesty, appreciate incitement that doesn't zero in on the penis. That being stated, there are a couple of undeniable differences that we'd be delinquent also since they are considered "a definitive" erogenous zones.

For ladies, a definitive erogenous zones comprise the areolas, clitoris, and G-spot. For men, these are the glans, frenulum, and prostate. As extraordinary as auxiliary erogenous zones may be, the vast majority of us actually need somewhat more to cross the end goal!

Erogenous Zones for Women FAQs

If you actually have consuming inquiries regarding how to utilize your erogenous zones, investigate our FAQs underneath.

What Number of Erogenous Zones Are There On The Female Body?

There isn't really a set number of erogenous zones for ladies. By and large, there are five to six essential erogenous zones, with quite a few expected optional zones.

The regions referenced in the erogenous zones graph above are auxiliary zones regular for the vast majority, however, every individual is different. You can figure out how to discover delight in another piece of your body contingent upon your encounters.

What Are a Woman's Most Erogenous Zones?

Your most erogenous regions are the ones generally associated with intercourse, including your areolas, clitoris, G-spot, cervix, and vaginal opening.

The most erogenous optional zones change from individual to individual. You'll just understand what you like by testing things out, so it's dependent upon you to discover what your most touchy zones are!

Are Women's Feet Erogenous Zones?

In spite of the fact that we did exclude them in the guide, numerous ladies do discover incitement of their feet pleasurable. Once more, this has to do with the sensitive inclination that can convert into sexual incitement.

Rubbing your feet is a decent method to build bloodstream and improve sentiments of excitement. You can even ask your accomplice to delicately grovel to you and toes, yet keep an eye out! Feet might be an erogenous zone for certain ladies yet demonstrate excessively sensitivity for other people.

When it comes to erogenous zones, it isn't about the pinches, stubs, and cuts. Here are some improbable joy focuses that are often disregarded.

Scalp

The scalp is brimming with sensitive spots, and even the smallest brush of the hair can send shivers through your body. To amp up the delight, run your fingernails delicately over the scalp, giving exceptional consideration to the space behind the ears and simply over the neck.

Remember about the hair. Delicate pulling can send influxes of delight through the body.

Ears

With touchy skin outwardly and several tactile receptors within, the ears top the rundown of erogenous zones for some individuals.

For some sexy aural activity that is certain to, if it's not too much trouble, attempt softly kissing, licking, or snacking your accomplice's ear cartilage. You can likewise exploit those tangible receptors by murmuring or softly blowing into their ear for all the more shivery feels.

Navel and Lower Stomach

Being hazardously near the private parts makes this region particularly stimulating. Utilize your tongue, fingertips, or even a plume to follow hovers around the navel and bother your way down and all around the stomach.

This is an incredible spot for some temperature play, so utilize an ice 3D square if your accomplice is into it.

Playing solo? Touch the region to get yourself in the mind-set.

Little of the Back (Sacrum)

It could have something to do with the way that the nerves in this segment of the spine are associated with the pelvis, or the weakness factor of being contacted from behind that makes this region so touchy.

Whatever it is, the smallest touch here can summon delight. Stimulate the region with a quill or your lips and tongue.

Feeling brave? Attempt an ice 3D square, a vibrator, or pinwheel for some tactile play.

Inward Arms and Armpits

Figure armpits can't be sexy? Two words: "Messy Dancing."

You realize that scene where Johnny runs the rear of his hand down Baby's arm, brushing her armpit?

She laughs from the outset, however, once she moves beyond the stimulate reaction, it's absolutely hot.

A light touch is all you require to turn the tickle to thoroughly stimulating. Run your fingertips, your tongue, or even a quill gradually along the internal arm to the armpit.

Internal Wrist

Home of the best point and not used to getting a ton of activity, the inward wrist is exceptionally touchy.

Stroke the skin with your fingertips while taking a gander at your accomplice interestingly from over the table, or anyplace else so far as that is concerned, when attempting to set the temperament.

As of now in the pains of enthusiasm? Take a stab at entwining your fingers with theirs and touch the skin on their internal wrists with your lips and the tip of your tongue.

Palm of Hands and Fingertips

The fingertips are the piece of the body's most sensitive to contact, and your palms aren't a long way behind. Spot your hand under theirs with your palm looking up, and stimulate their palm with your pointer.

If you need to up the closeness, keep in touch while you do it.

You can kick it up a billion scores by taking every one of their fingers into your mouth, individually, and sucking daintily.

Behind the Knee

This is another often ignored region that is unfathomably touchy to any sort of touch. It's even sensitive for a few.

Give the region some uncommon consideration during a back rub, or utilize your mouth and tongue there prior to stirring your way up or down the leg.

The Ones You May Have Suspected

A portion of these might be pretty self-evident, yet others may very well shock you.

Areola

Areola incitement illuminates a similar zone in the mind as the privates.

Start with a light touch, and anything goes here. Lips, tongue, a plume, or a little vibrator are only a couple of thoughts.

Follow around the areola prior to moving onto the areola and sucking, licking, and in any event, flicking. Blow or utilize an ice solid shape for some sexy cool.

If your accomplice likes it harsh, touch the areola with your teeth. More unpleasant still? Attempt areola braces.

Mouth and Lips

Kissing is a craftsmanship, and we propose utilizing every last trace of their lips and mouth as your canvas.

Follow the state of their lips with your tongue prior to moving to a moderate, wet kiss, or tenderly suck or snack on their base lip.

Fun truth: There are scientifically demonstrated medical advantages to kissing, so pucker up.

Neck

When it goes to the neck, even the smallest touch can make your whole body shiver.

Fold your arms over your accomplice, and run your fingernails along the rear of their neck, moving to the zone behind the ears prior to advancing around the front.

Proceed onward to delicately kissing the sides and front of the neck prior to working your way to the lips or traveling south where it's significantly more blazing.

Inward Thighs

The inward thighs are so delicate and very near a definitive erogenous zone that even only a touch can set your flanks burning.

Run your fingertips down the front of the thighs, gradually moving your direction internally while you kiss their lips, neck, and chest.

When you're prepared to get very close, cover the zone in delicate, wet kisses and licks.

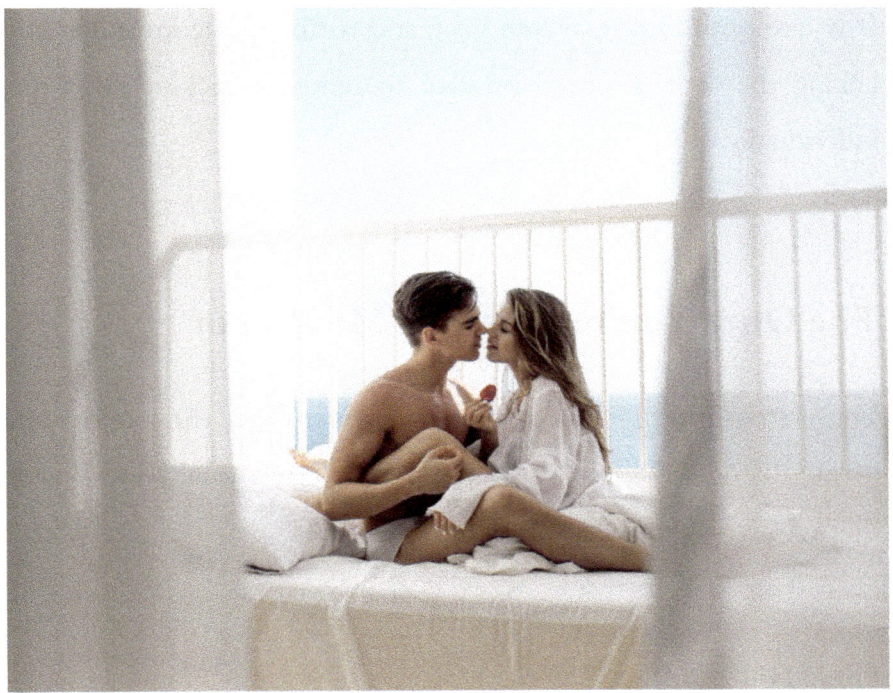

Lower Part of Feet and Toes

Weight focuses on the lower part of the feet can build bloodstream and upgrade sentiments of excitement when controlled perfectly.

Investigation with different weights when rubbing the feet, beginning light, and working your path more profound until you find what works.

If you're both into it, switch back and forth among kneading and licking the foot. Proceed onward to tenderly sucking each toe, individually.

The Ones You're Certainly Mindful of

These may appear to be pretty self-evident, yet the vaginal and penile districts contain various different erogenous zones inside them. How about we jump right in, will we?

Pubic Hill

The mons pubis, the plump hill simply over the clitoris, is wealthy in sensitive spots that are associated with the private parts. Rubbing the territory in a here and there movement can in a roundabout way animate the labia and clitoris.

If your accomplice is responsive to additional, proceed onward to kissing the zone, then utilize the tip of your tongue to lick your way down. If you're playing with yourself, back rub or vibe to up your excitement.

Clitoris

This little delight bud contains more than 8,000 sensitive spots and is covered by a hood. Tenderly take it between your file and center finger and slide it gradually in an all-over movement.

Need more? Utilize your fingers or a clitoral vibrator and rub your stub utilizing lightweight. Examination with bearing and beat to discover what feels best.

For some great tongue activity, start moderate and speed up and pressure.

A-Spot

The lower portion of the vaginal opening is loaded with sexually charged sensitive spots and home to the front fornix (A-spot).

Use fingers, a dildo, or penis to infiltrate the vagina, and spotlight tension on the front divider while sliding in and out.

G-Spot

The G-spot is a region fit for causing what's known as female discharge. Fingers or a bent G-spot vibrator are your smartest option for arriving at it.

With a decent measure of lube, turn your vibrator or finger upward toward the navel and move it in a "come here" movement.

Find what feels better and keep at it, permitting the sensation to fabricate.

Cervix

An individual should be completely stirred to appreciate cervical incitement, so foreplay is an unquestionable requirement.

Any profound entrance sex position can do it. Doggy style is a decent one that can be performed utilizing a tie on or ordinary dildo, as well. When you discover a profundity and movement that feels better, continue onward.

Cervical climaxes are like what's known as a full-body climax in tantric sex, so you're in for a treat if you can arrive.

Penile District

Glans

The glans penis is what's known as the head. Because of 4,000 sensitive spots, it's the most touchy piece of the penis.

Bother it by scouring your wet lips delicately over the plump head prior to utilizing the tip of your tongue around the edge. Next, bring the glans into your mouth, whirling your tongue around it.

A very much lubed hand can likewise do some incredible things.

Frenulum

This is the flexible bit of skin on the underside of the penis, where the pole meets the head. It's exceptionally delicate and the essential trigger of climaxes in individuals with penises.

Hands or Mouth

To get convenient with it, slide your lubed hand all over the pole, letting your thumb touch the F-spot. During a penis massage, ensure your tongue gives additional consideration to this problem area.

Prepuce

The prepuce is loaded up with sensitive spots that really upgrade joy for those with uncircumcised penises. This meager layer of skin gives the occasion to blend it up for different sensations during a handwork or penis massage.

You can let it float over the penis and organs with each stroke or delicately withdraw it to zero in on the exposed F-spot and head. Be delicate and use lube.

Scrotum and Balls

The coin tote is loaded up with super-delicate nerves holding on to be delighted in. Tenderly back rub the balls during a sensual caress, handwork, or while stroking off.

Up the joy by demonstrating the scrotal raphe some affection. This is the crease that runs down the focal point of the scrotum. Run your finger tenderly all over the raphe while stroking off, or let your tongue do something amazing for the crease when performing oral.

Perineum

This touchy fix of skin lies between the scrotum and butt. You can arrive at this hot southern objective from practically any position on yourself or another person. Reach past the sack during a handwork or penis massage and rub it, or reach between the legs during minister sex. Utilize your knuckle to apply pressure while sliding it to and fro. Do it as discharge approaches for a staggering peak.

Prostate

This pecan estimated organ sits at the base of the penis and can prompt ground-breaking, sheet-turning climaxes. You can just arrive at the P-spot by means of B-town, so an all around lubed finger or prostate vibrator works best. Tenderly supplement your finger or vibrator several crawls into the rectum, applying strain to the front divider. When you locate the correct move, keep at it. Stroke or suck the penis simultaneously for greatest joy.

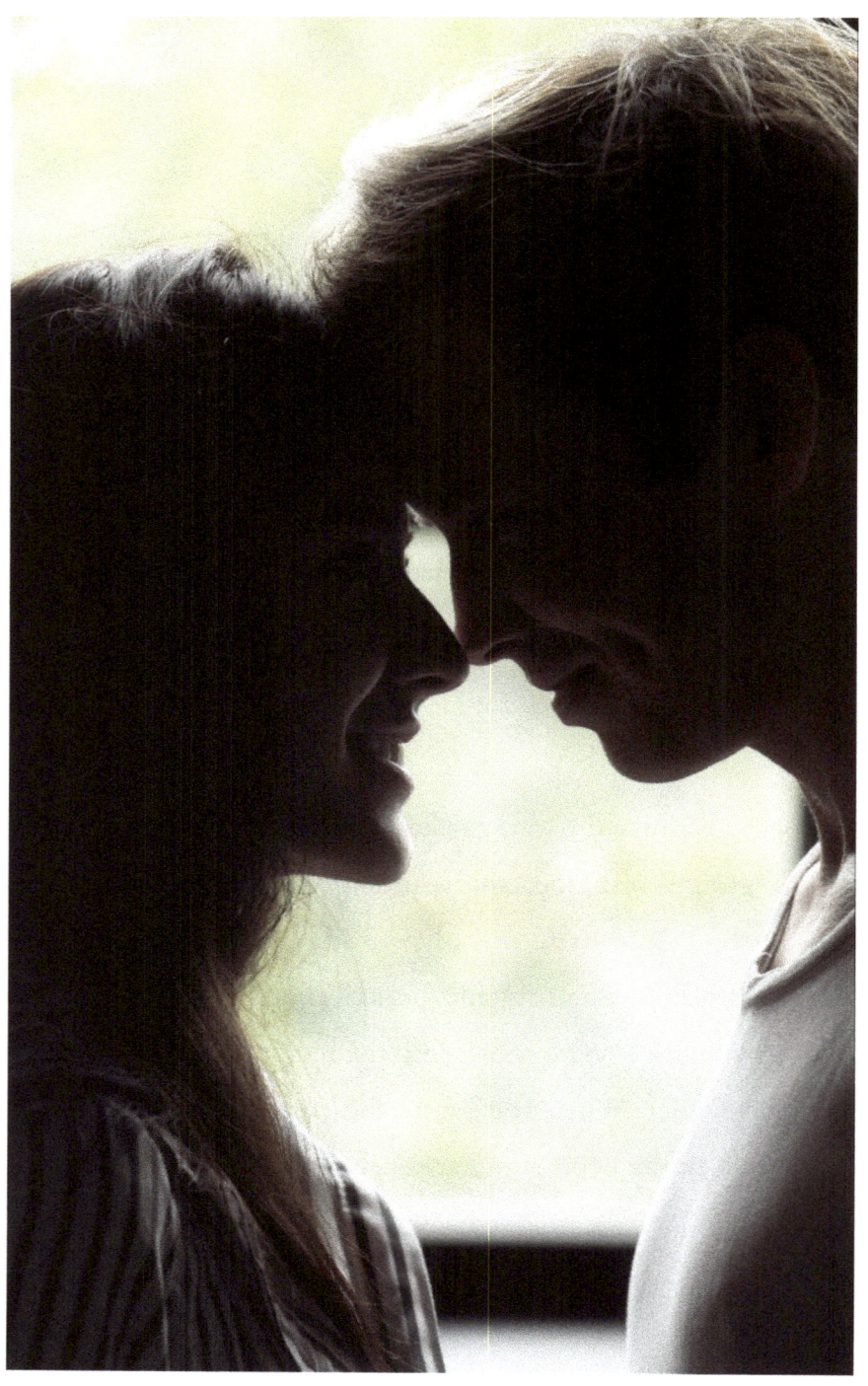

CHAPTER 3. SPIRITUAL PHASE OF SEXUAL ENERGY

Carefulness about sex through those early hundreds of years is justifiable. Prior to present day medication, maybe a fourth of all ladies in the long run passed on in labor. No powerful prophylactic was accessible.

Youngsters conceived without any father present were social outcasts. A non-virgin lady would be unable to actually discover a spouse and required monetary help. Sexually sent illnesses had no fix. Sexual inclinations were thought to decrease individuals to the degree of a creature. On numerous fronts, sex was believed to be, and indeed was, risky.

In any case, why has religion remained violently sex-negative even today? Rehashed contemplates show that the more strict individuals are, the more contradicted to sex they will in general be.

An almost insane strict operation position to sex—for instance, the enrollment of a huge number of American duty dollars to advance sexual forbearance broadly and universally—makes one can't help thinking about what is truly going on.

There is no simple representation of this strict interest. To clarify social mentalities is difficult in the best of cases and, maybe, unimaginable in a period of fast change, similar to our own.

Yale history specialist John Boswell contended that Christianity has essentially followed common mores with respect to sexual issues. A long way from establishing the tone, Christianity tended simply to give it an otherworldly endorsement. Today, when a really religious conversation of homosexuality has emerged, Christianity faces a novel test: to figure out sexual issues philosophically, notwithstanding mushrooming new proof.

Truth be told, such figuring out has just been finished. Religious contentions to authentic sexual variety—scriptural, verifiable, organic, clinical, mental, sociological, anthropological, moral—are there for any individual who needs them. However, the religions won't change their educating. Why so? The causes are numerous, complex, and entwined. A posting of likely ones will reveal some insight into this problem.

• Ignorance is a central point. Sexuality has been a subject of study for scarcely a century. Sigmund Freud's infamous accentuation on sex was not an individual idiosyncrasy, but rather an impression of the maturing interest of his day. In the previous century, we have become familiar with sex than during all of earlier human history. Sexual direction, transsexualism, transvestism, intersexuality—these subjects never fit into customary thoughts of sex, yet today they are known as generally normal, non-neurotic, characteristic varieties.

Religionists are up to speed short of needing to confront these issues, and, notwithstanding their profound good commitment to give equipped otherworldly authority, numerous individuals from the church basically don't have the foggiest idea, or are reluctant to concede, the as of late learned realities.

• The ground-breaking feelings that encompass sexuality are another factor. Feelings of cloud thinking. If, in all honesty, the heart as a rule governs the head. So some strict pioneers—particularly seniors, who will generally hold the persuasive positions, however, who experienced childhood in previous ages with profoundly engrained prohibitive sexual perspectives—may really be humanly unequipped for rising above their biases. In addition, more youthful ministry additionally experienced childhood in sexual constraint. It will take ages before comfort with sex gets regular of our general public.

• Emotional rebuilding of the human mind is a moderate cycle. Profound mental recuperating often requires long periods of psychotherapy. However, the feeling partner loaded social changes that attack our period have come rapidly—separate, synthetic contraception, racial equity, ladies' privileges, access for the crippled, gay freedom, transsexual and intersex freedom, gay marriage, the Internet, the breakdown of public limits, the development of a worldwide network, and psychological warfare.

The human mind isn't worked to support such quick fire attack. By any verifiable norm, the accomplishments of sexual freedom, regardless of whether it ended today, would stay exceptional. Indeed, then, it isn't out of the ordinary that individuals as a rule or their religions will change their sexual perspectives rapidly.

Blame is another factor. Sexual investigation is an ordinary part of pre-adulthood. In that investigation, numerous individuals do things that later burden their still, small voices—particularly men and particularly with respect to homosexual play.

My human sexuality class in provincial, Bible-Belt Georgia, for instance, quite often rates as obvious, without banter, that equivalent sex experimentation is a typical aspect of their way of life. Yet, given the cultural and strict blame encompassing such sex acts, grown-up devotees, changed over and humble, are probably going to wage a fight against sexual "sins," their own and everybody else's.

The way that even these genuine adherents had once "fallen" gives individual confirmation of the need to carefully contradict poisonous homosexuality.

• Reaction arrangement—the Freudian safeguard instrument whereby one restricts in others what one faculty yet can't concede in oneself—additionally happens in different ways. Carl Jung noticed that homosexual individuals will generally be profoundly touchy. So they are probably going to be overrepresented in the service.

Assessments of homosexual Catholic clerics range from 30 to 60 percent and then some. Because of the all-male structure of the Catholic organization, this occurrence of homosexuality is presumably higher than that among the non-Catholic churches.

In any case, regardless of the accepted prerequisite of marriage for Protestant clergymen, the occurrence of homosexuality among them is likewise prone to be high.

Additionally, an ongoing report proposed that "heterosexual" men who become all the more sexually stimulated by homosexual erotic entertainment likewise will generally score higher than others on a size of homophobia. Generally speaking, then, some pastorate most likely contradicts homosexuality because they can't acknowledge the propensity in themselves.

• Changing sexual mores shake the very establishments of Western development, so dread additionally catalyzes strict pioneers in their opposition to change. Such change is inalienable in the "sexual upset," and such change is epic, so opposition to it isn't entirely unreasonable. In peril of verifiable change lie the standard of man controlled society, the connection boat of man and lady, the thoughts of gentility and manliness, the magically amazing and monetarily hindering heterosexual wedding, the famous comprehension of marriage, and the Norman-Rockwellian fantasy of family. The danger likewise incorporates the fictionalized energy of "free sex" released, the intensity of sentiment to weaken the hard working attitude, and the loss of simple legislative authority over individuals because they love.

The development toward a worldwide network—based on the adage of "human rights" and aware of all people groups and societies yet controlled for monetary objectives by global companies—is another entrapped measurement of this complicated situation. Under confusing conditions like these, it is justifiable that strict pioneers would incline toward traditionalism and, inept as anybody to limit the chronicled patterns, would zero in on people, their private sex lives, and their dread ridden relationship with God. Obviously and sadly, strict confidence isn't sufficiently able to permit that everything individuals could act naturally and still live respectively in harmony, bliss, and shared regard. We are as yet unequipped for considering a really new world request.

• Philosophically, too, the base has dropped out of Western development. Revolutionary postmodernism ruins the very ideas of truth and goodness, and moderate postmodernism has, at all, exhibited the difficulty of moving toward these conventional standards. No agreement at all on epistemology or morals exists in our day. Indeed, even the chance of right knowledge has been— self-conflictingly—contended unflinchingly. Nobody—with the exception of, I accept, Bernard Lonergan—visualizes a trustworthy exit from this problem. Consequently, religion's simple case to know reality from God and to declare the great shows up as a fiction from a past period. Regardless, better to have a questionable moral educating than none by any stretch of the imagination.

So religion holds to its conventional position. This propensity is obtrusive in Roman Catholicism, which keeps on demanding that for each situation, sex must be available to origination. Different religions are not as express in their educating, but rather sensible investigation of their opposition to sexual varieties because of an alleged "complementarity of the sexes" prompts a similar first reason. Hence, for the need of an intelligible other option, religion demands the floundering the norm.

• Appeal to the Bible ought not to continue opposition to lesbian and gay relationships, yet it does. As pertinently as chronicled research is ever liable to do, scriptural grant shows that perceived in their unique semantic, recorded, and social settings, the scriptural writings were not tending to the inquiries of our day and didn't denounce same-sex acts as such in their day. Despite the fact that not all permit so clear an end, in the extremely least, a legit individual must concede that there is not kidding question about the significance of those writings. This uncertainty should support sexual variety. Standard and long-standing strict standards apply in such cases.

For instance, Catholic instructing holds that it isn't on the whole correct to force an ethical weight on an individual if the requirement for that weight is sketchy: Lex dubia not obligat: A dicey law has no coupling power. Also, Baptists advocate "soul opportunity," the privilege of each adherent to actually hold their own understanding of the Bible and its prerequisites. However, neither of these religions cuts slack for lesbian and gay individuals. Clearly, similarly as ownership is nine-tenths of the law, so settled good educating exceeds ongoing understanding. In this way, for all the reasons previously noted and contrary to their own customary moral standards, religions keep on easily contradict homosexuality.

• Blatant human backwardness, out and out evil, is likewise a factor that ought not to be neglected. It shows itself in scapegoating: the simple fault of lesbians and gays for all the ills of society; in a deceitful, however politically practical play on individuals' feelings of dread for winning races and continuing abusive political plans; and in the rewarding appeal to homophobia in strict gathering pledges endeavors. A comparable dynamic, less intentionally blamable, is employable inside ministers' and hierarchs' feelings of dread of parting gatherings and entire strict bodies over a questionable change in genuinely charged sexual approach.

• Finally, reasonableness necessitates that we permit the kindness of the individuals who restrict homosexuality. Without a doubt and lamentably, numerous strict pioneers genuinely accept that sexual varieties are destructive, off-base, heathen, and evil.

Their reasons may be an un-unsure combination of those recorded above or others that relate to summed up strict devotion, for example, confidence in a specific religion, the voice of the pope, or the expression of the Bible, the Koran, or the Book of Mormon. Despite the fact that others—myself included—might consider them to be as a fiction of visually impaired conviction, the honorability of their profound duty must be credited.

Clearly, generally, strict conversation of homosexuality is certainly not a sane undertaking. I know no other subject whose simple notice can make a few people lose all point of view, capitulate to amygda-loid rage, and go bonkers.

The inescapable difference in strict convictions, decisions, and perspectives will be difficult. While the moderate cycle of progress goes on, otherworldly pioneers—liberal, addressing, legit, and great willed—need to fashion another vision of the relationship between sexuality and otherworldliness. Such a dream will give traditionalist religionists a rational and moral other option. This they can grasp in the great soul when they at long last start to relinquish their sex cynicism. To such a dream, this article turns indeed.

The Human as Body, Mind, and Soul

In their anxiety to restrict sexual experience, Augustine and Aquinas were right: Sexual experience involves a transitory loss of judiciousness. Yet, with more significant mental mindfulness, the insight of our age affirms that such a brief misfortune may be acceptable.

The psychoanalytic term that could apply is "relapse in the administration of the self image." Sometimes it is helpful to encounter a break from our too-potent logic. Such "relapse" permits our psychological structures to pull together in a more beneficial arrangement: one stage in reverse for two stages forward. Similarly as a required excursion lets us re-visitation of regular day-to-day existence with another standpoint, in this way, as well, a rest from our over supported and over-intellectualized interests can carry another feeling of miracle to every day living.

To be human is to be ever turning out to be. For the duration of our lives we make ourselves. In the end every one of us will be simply the unparalleled version.

Our turning out to be relied upon a shifting equilibrium in the different aspects of our make up. As an interruption that gives new life, sex can give an event to shift our inward equilibrium. In any case, what does this shift have to do with otherworldly development?

Religion has generally considered the human being as a blend of body and soul. Also, brain science talks about the body and psyche. The difference between psyche and soul does not merit tending to now. The two ideas are adequately fluffy that looking at them would be a squandered exertion. All things considered, this much remaining parts clear: A two-section model of the human being is excessively straightforward. There is all the more going on in internal human experience—soul or brain—than only a certain something.

In his significant work, Insight: A Study of Human Understanding, Bernard Lonergan discusses two features of the psyche. The one continually asks us into new boondocks and toward additional development; different looks for, rather, the solace and security of a steady the norm.

Lonergan calls the principal purposeful cognizance of the human soul, and the other, mind. Hence, he extends a three-sided model of the human being: body, mind, and soul.

Soul is oneself rising above element of the human brain. We experience it most fundametally as a miracle, wonder, stunningness. It prompts us to know, to act naturally mindful, and even to know about our mindfulness. Its very nature is "question"— outward-looking dynamism, crude interest, that would see always and more and incorporate perpetually, and that's just the beginning.

Open-finished in its domain, its optimal objective is all that there is to know and adore. It is, indeed, that by which we do come to know and cherish. It manages our marvel, our scrutinizing, our judging, and our picking.

Outfitted to grasp the universe—even as, in the ideal, we would need to comprehend everything about everything and in the process become one with everything—it is an inherent homing gadget for our life's journey. It "knows" what is needed for completeness, unity, lucidness, solidarity—similarly as, when we pose an inquiry, we foresee what sort of answer will fulfill our inquiry.

In like manner, it "detects" when we skirt off course—similarly as without really knowing the right answer, we perceive when we're given a "bait and switch" and a proposed answer doesn't generally address our inquiry. Following the lead of this inward manual for the degree that we are capable, we would keep on evolving, move, and develop until we arrived at the totality of the positive development that is conceivable in our specific life circumstances.

This internal mental drive makes them live in a universe of understandings and love, of implications and qualities, of thoughts and goals, of dreams and temperances.

Differently named, these issues are plainly otherworldly; they are not of reality. Because of this component of our brains, staying right where we will be, we can rise above existence. We can get a handle on abstracts, for example, $a2 + b2 = c2$ and $t' = t\sqrt{1-v2/c2}$—which apply all over the place and consistently. We can have encounters—mystery—in which we appear to achieve solidarity, all things considered. This component of our psyches is appropriately called soul.

It is that because of which Genesis says that we are made in the "picture and similarity" of God, and the Psalmist says that we are made "somewhat less than the heavenly attendants." It is that because of which Saint Augustine said in petition, "Ruler, you have made us for yourself, and our hearts are eager till they rest in you." It is what makes us people, to a limited extent, profound creatures, as opposed to beast creatures or lifeless things.

Without ever expressly discussing God or of a relationship with God, I have been portraying an aspect of our psyches that is profound. If I am right in this manner, this very part of our psyches is the premise of human otherworldliness.

Because of it, we know marvel and amazement, we question our reality, we ponder the stars, we connect in adoration—and envisioning the solution to our every inquiry and anticipating the satisfaction to our most profound longings, we imagine God. The human soul is the genuine establishment of all otherworldliness. Religious contemplations are optional; they are subsidiary.

To the degree that we permit the human soul to control our living, to the degree that we incorporate its urgings always into the very structure of our being, we develop profoundly; we become more otherworldly. Be that as it may, this self-rising above measurement isn't entirely there is to our brains.

There is likewise mind. It underpins the out going soul; it "houses" the soul. In any case, by a similar token, the mind likewise restricts the soul.

The best deterrent to our otherworldly development is ourselves. Despite the fact that our spirits would take off, features of our brains forestall such self-amazing quality.

For reasons additionally incorporated with our being, we can't be completely liberal, we limit our miracle and wonder, we dread to strike out on new undertakings, we egotistically go to just to ourselves. Our self-restricting self-protection limits our potential for limitless development.

Clinicians and instructors work to let loose the restricting parts of oneself. These experts assist us with mending our previous damages, quit any pretense of putrefying feelings of disdain, improve relational relationships, set aside counter beneficial safeguards.

The focal point of such recuperating is feelings, recollections, pictures, and propensities for character. All these settle on up what Lonergan decisions mind.

Subsequently, there is a pull a lot within us. The inclination to develop and the desire to deteriorate are at battle inside us—maybe like the "soul" and "substance" about which Saint Paul composed.

The objective of development is to coordinate these inward powers and to let soul start to lead the pack until, through rehashed self-change, our entire being—body, mind, and soul—moves amicably in one course. Such is the way of otherworldly development.

Perceived from a mental perspective—that is, a humanistic or naturalistic, not yet a philosophical perspective—profound development results through the cycle of reconciliation of the human soul.

The Component of Otherworldly Development

Presently it comes clear what a delay in routine has to do with profound development. It is now and then valuable to break out of our routinized world to permit our spirits to start to lead the pack.

This doesn't involve going on retreat to permit God into our lives—as though God were not as of now continually working through regular causes in and around us and, as Christianity would add, through the powerful gift of the Holy Spirit, who has been immersed our hearts. On my arrangement, otherworldliness is, fairly, most importantly, a promise to delivering oneself rising above human soul that is ever as of now a piece wondrous being.

Appropriately, as reflective practice, sex can likewise be a way toward individual—and, therefore, profound—combination. By moving us out of our workaday world and into a more innovative mental space, similar to contemplation, sexual encounters can cultivate the change of the mind. Such mental mending is the natural instrument of otherworldly development.

While a previous age stressed opposition among body and soul, contemporary mental mindfulness accentuates mix—because it improves humanity, and iron-willed concealment doesn't. This mental exercise is certain.

Weight cooker-like, suppressed emotions, and tendencies definitely break out, yet with conscious consideration, internal powers can be uncovered, perceived, and capably diverted into pathways of self-improvement. Along these lines, rather than endeavoring to sequester sex, to limit, control, and limit it, our age would perceive sexual variety, and for each situation help body, mind, and soul go into an interesting, life-improving association.

Rather than imagining the profound ideal to escape from the actual body and world, our age would discover otherworldly development through close to home satisfaction in the body—in a life of marvel, stunningness, trustworthiness, appreciation, love, administration, and kindness. The other-common otherworldliness of a previous age is today offering an approach to "incarnational otherworldliness," a this-common way of completeness and combination.

Allowed that one aspect of human completeness is the human soul, individual combination involves ipso facto expanding realization of our profound potential. Instead of contradict sex, contemporary accentuation would utilize sex to inspire and incorporate this potential. This impact can happen on two levels: substantial and clairvoyant.

Real Gets to the Soul

Tibetan Buddhism has since quite a while ago utilized actual sexual excitement to accomplish otherworldly encounters. We know this convention as Tantric sex. In our own general public interest in "sensual back rub" is promoting this equivalent methodology.

It utilizes full-body knead, including sexual incitement, however, without climax, to initiate extraordinary and delayed conditions of physiological excitement. Particularly when joined by profound breathing activities, this excitement can initiate significantly changed conditions of cognizance, which, as hallucinogenic medications utilized strictly or psychotherapeutically, encourage the rebuilding of the mind.

Comparative reports are made about karezza, delayed non-orgasmic sex, which was spearheaded in the Oneida Colony and later promoted by Dr. Alice Stockman. Indeed, even performance sex, often shockingly, evokes pictures, recollections, and longings that offer new alternatives forever. In humans, for whom the cerebrum is the biggest sex organ, climax is indivisibly connected to the operations of the psyche.

Because the body is the establishment of the mind, any sexual excitement slackens up the mind. The unwinding that sexual excitement requires opens up the psyche.

Dream regularly goes with sexual excitement: pictures, recollections, and feelings ascend out of the mind. This purge of the mind opens the best approach to individual change. Hence, sexual excitement can fill in as an admittance to the soul through the body—similarly as other, more norm, body-focused otherworldly practices do, for example, fasting, lack of sleep, yoga, ceremonial stances, development, and sacrosanct intoxicants.

Mystic Gets to the Soul

A passing sexual experience can in some cases be a gainful encounter—the unbelievable end of the week tryst that leaves the two players appreciative for each another and reestablished confidence in life.

All things considered, fair and square of mind, sexual excitement has its most impressive impact when combined with sentiment and continuous relationship.

The passionate intensity of relationships is unbelievable. Darlings relentlessly challenge each other as they run forward and backward in a dance of ongoing trade-offs and changes, a few stages invited and others stood up to. Some of the time, the intensity of relational relationships can be hazardous; be that as it may, somewhat for each situation, they get into the mind.

Beginning to look all starry-eyed and being enamored are energizing and upsetting encounters. When individuals are infatuated, from their minds come spilling out recollections, delights, and fears—just as expectations and plans: the fantasies and guarantees of sweethearts, the implications and qualities, the thoughts and standards that are the signs of the human soul. This mystic change turns over rich mental soil and clears a path for new development. With the breakdown of constant examples of conduct and reaction comes the chance of reconfiguring the self in a more beneficial structure. In this sense, individuals in cherishing relationships are "beneficial for one another."

Sex can be utilized to encourage self-extraordinary experience. Having intercourse allures darlings into dreaming dreams and making guarantees: Human sex connects with the mind, which, thus, delivers the human soul.

Carrying a purified brain to sex additionally changes sex itself. Therefore, contrasted with the uninformed, individuals who contemplate routinely can be all the more actually occupied with a sexual experience.

They can move toward a collaboration with the lucidity of the center, knowing why they are there; with force of activity, being completely present to each development, contact, and signal; with passionate attunement, streaming in synchronize with the accomplice; with the responsiveness of quality, going to suddenly to the next; and with significant identification, ending up in the other and the other in themselves.

While the normal meditator carries a more extravagant self to the sexual experience, the substantial and clairvoyant impacts of the experience additionally further intensify the meditator's very own quality. This correspondence makes a snowballing impact. Different frameworks plan to expand individual—and now relational—incorporation. Bodies, minds, and spirits stream in the rising above, ever-restoring course that is controlled by the open-finished dynamism of the human soul itself. A unitive encounter—a feeling of unity with oneself, the other, and the universe—may here and there result.

This is to state, in sexual sharing or in reflection on it, one can know a snapshot of otherworldly rapture.

As does each "strict experience," this second assists with encouraging change in the mind, opening onto the chance of still further encounters of self-change. In this style, adoring sex can turn into a way to otherworldly satisfaction.

The Ideal and the Genuine in Context

Notwithstanding, my practical feeling of life necessitates that I add a qualification. It must be reviewed that sex is frequently a somewhat mundane occasion. Individuals, for the most part, wind up appreciating sex, not because it can make the way for mystery yet for either more commonplace explanation. Similarly as with otherworldliness itself, we should be mindful so as not to admire sex.

It is often short of what it is supposed to be. Sex is, all things considered, a human issue, and, as a general rule, human undertakings fall into the dim reach, not into dark or white.

In any case, sex and otherworldliness can be coordinated. They can commonly improve one another. Be that as it may, as the cozy relationship between sexuality and otherworldliness turns into a subject of famous conversation, misdirecting oversimplifications arise. I clarified the inalienable relationship of sexuality to otherworldliness based on an aspect of our human cosmetics—to be specific, the open-finished, self-rising above, dynamic, and normatively organized human soul.

Allowed this agreement, few out of every odd sexual experience is profoundly helpful. In itself, obviously, as sheer sensation, sex has a sorcery. In any case, this simply physical and passionate fervor isn't oneself rising above the miracle of the human soul. An extraordinary sexual excitement prompts otherworldly satisfaction.

Medications can actuate profoundly valuable changed conditions of awareness, and numerous indigenous strict customs—also Christianity's utilization of fellowship wine on a vacant stomach—use hallucinogenics for this reason; however, individuals likewise use drugs in the city and end up in oppressing addictions.

Likewise, sex can be utilized for profound development, however, it can likewise be utilized for idealism. In its own particular manner, sex can likewise turn into a compulsion. It would be an exacerbated deception to accept that a voracious quest for sex has profound development as its thought process or its probable result.

The otherworldly way follows a scarcely discernible difference. It is the thin door of which Jesus talked, the razor edge that the bodhisattva must walk.

If a previous age tumbled off the edge into an other-common outrageous, pushing a profound satisfaction that necessary the refusal of sex, our own age will in general tumble off the edge into a this-common extraordinary, disregarding the otherworldly and promoting the estimation of actual delight.

Finding and communicating an equilibrium isn't anything but difficult to do. However, more awful than missing the equilibrium is to not endeavor to discover it. Joining of sexuality and otherworldliness may require some experimentation, and en route one may commit a few errors.

One just expectations that we as a whole have the great sense not to commit unsalvageable errors, for example, undesirable pregnancies, hopeless sexually sent infections, broken hearts, or shameful disloyalties of serious duties. I treat the joining of sexuality and otherworldliness in detail in Sex and the Sacred.

The Reconciliation of Sexuality and Otherworldliness

Otherworldliness is a journey. Made out of body, mind, and soul, we live pulled in numerous ways. The test every day is to seek after another equilibrium as life unavoidably changes and proceeds onward.

The way into the equilibrium is attunement to our own soul, for the soul holds a dream of solidarity, a direction toward greatness, and a wellspring of shrewdness that are past our purposeful control.

For that very explanation—because our own soul appears to work from past ourselves, because we are more than our little, conceptualized selves—individuals will generally ascribe otherworldly encounters to things outside of themselves, most regularly, to "God."

I have credited otherworldliness to a part creatures. Appropriately comprehended, this methodology prompts no solipsism, self-centeredness, selfism, heathen humanism, agnostic naturalism, or nearsighted insignificance—as pundits affirm—for our spirits are basically friendly, outfitted to the universe, arranged to all that is valid and acceptable. Constancy to the human soul couldn't yet lead godward.

One preferred position of this methodology is that it effectively clarifies the cozy relationship between otherworldliness and sexuality—and numerous different aspects of human living, too. Another bit of leeway is that it counters the very long term humiliation of Christianity—the religion that trusts God became tissue yet has regarded the substance as disgraceful.

CHAPTER 4. SEX TOYS FOR PLEASURE

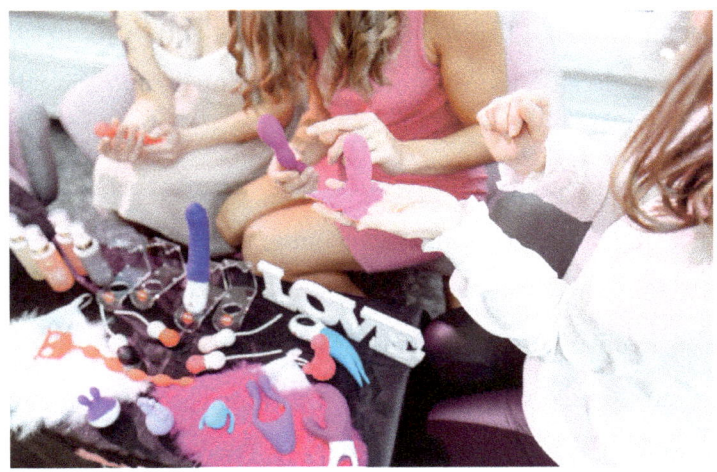

For some individuals, the main sexual partner we have is ourselves, and masturbation is the manner in which we become more acquainted with our sexual selves. As we contact ourselves, we investigate our bodies, find new sensations, and attempt various methods. Masturbation is a blessing, a demonstration of confidence. Individuals jerk off with various goals and for various reasons: to have a climax, to fantasize, to liquefy away pressure, to help nod off (or awaken), or to feel an association with your own body. Utilizing a toy while you stroke off is a decent method to find out about your body and your sexuality, reinforce and tone your pelvic muscles, zest up your daily practice, and investigate another action.

Self-Discovery For Better Sex

Most young men start to stroke off when they hit pubescence; their first erection, wet dream, and masturbation meeting are on the whole soul changing experiences in our general public. When they are youthful adults, they've investigated how their penis works and have jerked off to climax. Then again, numerous young ladies don't have an equal encounter. A young lady's first clitoral hard-on isn't actually a typical subject in mainstream society. Also, ladies aren't urged to grasp their sexual bodies similarly that men are. Accordingly, numerous ladies don't jerk off routinely or have never stroked off. This twofold standard places ladies at an incredible detriment in their sexual development, and they frequently grow up with sensations of irresoluteness, blame, disarray, or disgrace about their own bodies.

For a lady who's never jerked off, a sex toy like a vibrator is an extraordinary method to acquaint her with the thought. On the off chance that she feels bashful about contacting herself or shaky about what to do, a vibrator can loan the aiding, um, hand she needs. Additionally, for ladies who've never had a climax or who experience difficulty arriving at orgasm, a vibrator is regularly suggested by sex advisors and doctors. Despite your sex, self-disclosure shouldn't end once you become explicitly dynamic. At the point when individuals approach me for tips on the best way to improve as a sweetheart, I have one recommendation for everybody: jerk off. Truth be told: The more you engage in sexual relations with yourself, the better you'll be at having intercourse with your partner. Self-information is the way to sexual wellbeing, prosperity, and joy. Furthermore, the more you think about your own body—what you like, what you don't, what feels better, what doesn't, what turns you on, what kills you—the more you can impart to your partner.

Utilizing a toy while you jerk off is likewise a decent method to evaluate something new. Maybe you're keen on testing—with utilizing a vibrator, trying out a cock ring, or investigating anal penetration. Whatever it will be, it very well might be something you're interested about, however you're not prepared to examine it or give it a shot with your partner. That is alright. You don't need to share each sexual craving you have with your partner immediately. All things being equal, check it out during an independent meeting, and perceive how you like it. Maybe you'll choose to hush up about it, saving it for self-pleasuring events. Or on the other hand you may find that you like it such a lot of that you need to impart it to your partner.

Sexual Exercise for Better Health

Masturbation isn't simply fun, it's in reality bravo! Similarly as we realize that activity is useful for our bodies and decreases the danger of specific conditions and diseases, practicing our sexual life structures is additionally significant. In particular, practicing the pubococcygeus muscles (otherwise called the PC muscles) assumes a major job in people sexual wellbeing. The PC muscles run from the pubic issue that remains to be worked out tailbone, supporting the uterus, bladder, and gut. For people the same, these muscles contract arbitrarily when you are explicitly stimulated and musically during orgasm. By conditioning and fortifying the PC muscles through exercise, men can improve prostate wellbeing, figure out how to control and postpone discharge, control incontinence, keep up better erections, and experience greater affectability during sex.

For ladies, the PC muscles can be pushed, debilitated, or decayed from heftiness, during pregnancy and labor, after a time of sexual forbearance, or similarly as a component of the maturing cycle. By practicing and fortifying your PC muscles, you can improve in line with the sentiments in your pelvic zone, expanding your affectability and responsiveness. The activities will likewise condition the pelvic muscles, making them more adaptable and more responsive to pleasurable sensations.

Ladies who routinely practice their PC and pelvic muscles report it encourages them:

• Maintain urinary plot wellbeing

• Prevent or control incontinence

• Prepare for pregnancy and labor

• Achieve more noteworthy affectability during sex

• Have expanded joy during clitoral stimulation and vaginal and anal entrance

• Have better, more controlled orgasms

Kegel practices were named for the doctor who initially promoted the hypothesis of practicing PC muscles. You can do the activities resting, sitting, or standing, and doing them during masturbation will build blood stream to the privates and increment your excitement. Likewise with other exercise regimens, this ought to be performed every day for best outcomes. In the event that your muscles appear to be drained from the outset, don't stress—that is typical. The harder the activities are to accomplish for you, the less conditioned your PC muscles are, and the more you need an exercise. Utilize your good judgment, and don't try too hard in the first place; in the event that you experience any agony while doing them, see a specialist.

To find your PC muscles, envision that you are attempting to quit peeing (or while you are peeing, you can really stop the progression of pee). The muscles you agreement to stop the stream are your PC muscles. You can likewise slide a finger inside your vagina and attempt to crush your finger with your muscles. Whenever you've discovered the PC muscles, take some full breaths. Agreement the muscles and hold the compression for a couple of moments. At that point loosen up the muscles. Start to add one moment to the daily practice, and see whether you can stir your way as long as 10 seconds of withdrawal followed by 10 seconds of unwinding. You can do these in arrangements of ten a few times each day. For best outcomes, ensure you're disconnecting the PC muscle. Try not to hold your breath or agreement your stomach or different muscles.

Vaginal Exercise: Try Ben-Wa Balls, Stone Eggs, and Barbells

A few people accept that doing PC muscle practices with something inside the vagina (or in the anus for men) delivers better outcomes since you're working the muscles against some opposition. There are a few items planned particularly for Kegel works out.

Huge egg-molded toys made of cleaned jade, onyx, and other characteristic stones can be utilized by ladies to practice your PC muscles. You slide a very much lubed egg into your vagina, at that point work on getting your muscles around it. Since it's both thick and substantial, it gives all the more a test to the muscles. When the muscles

101

are more grounded, you can do the activities holding up. More modest and lighter than stone eggs, Ben-Wa balls are two balls on a string normally made of plastic or silicone. They are a decent starter for individuals threatened by the size and weight of the egg. Eggs and Ben-Wa balls ought not be utilized anally.

Heavier however not as thick as eggs, vaginal free weights are suggested by doctors, sexologists, and specialists for Kegel works out. The Kegelcisor and Betty's Vaginal Barbell (planned by masturbation master and sexologist Betty Dodson) are weighty metal dildos that are comparative in plan: They are around 7 inches (18 cm) long, weigh almost a pound, and have diverse measured balls on one or the flip side. You start by working on cinching down on the bigger ball, at that point graduate to the more modest one as your muscle tone improves; a few activities call for you to get the muscle while hauling the hand weight out of your vagina. The Natural Contours Energie is a comparative item, aside from it has a plastic covering over metal and a smooth surface without balls. Every one of the three can be utilized anally, yet with incredible alert, since they don't have erupted bases. At the point when the exercise is finished, the free weights, Ben-Wa balls, and stone egg can likewise be utilized as sex toys, only for joy.

Pleasure in Partnership Gets an Assist

Sex toys are intended for joy, and your sexual coexistence can profit by them from numerous points of view. Despite the fact that toys have progressed significantly since they were considered "conjugal guides," one thing stays valid: They can be issue solvers. Low drive is perhaps the most well-known issues that ladies face, particularly as they get more seasoned. For ladies who experience difficulty getting stirred, a vibrator can help kick the gathering off. For men, erectile brokenness and untimely discharge are two of the most widely recognized issues. Penis siphons can assist you with getting an erection; a cock ring can assist you with keeping a more grounded erection, postpone discharge, and draw out intercourse.

Quite possibly the most widely recognized grievances I get with ladies is that there isn't sufficient foreplay before intercourse. When all is said in done, it takes ladies additional time than men to get stirred. In the event that you engage in sexual relations before you're appropriately heated up, your body in a real sense isn't prepared: The private parts aren't completely engorged, and the vagina hasn't greased up and extended. A few ladies who experience torment during intercourse basically haven't given their bodies sufficient opportunity to fire up. A wide range of sex toys, including dildos and vibrators, can be utilized to encourage the excitement cycle. They can help make foreplay fun and perky, loosen up you, and get you in the mind-set. What's more, if your partner is exceptional, entrance with a toy that is somewhat more modest than him is an extraordinary method to get ready.

Sex toys can likewise give you an "additional arrangement of hands" in the room, permitting you to do a few things (or be in a few spots) immediately! Suppose you could give her vaginal entrance, clitoral stimulation, and anal delight all the while. You can with a butt plug, a vibrator, or a dildo to take care of you. At the point when the ideal situation for intercourse implies you can't arrive at different pieces of her body, a vibrator can be there for you. Consider the possibility that you need to play with his penis, balls, and areolas simultaneously. Areola cinches and a little vibrator will help you cover all his problem areas.

I like to consider sex toys as instruments for development: They grow your sexual collection. Probably the best thing about sex toys is that they can help you move away from an intercourse- consistently model of sex. Intercourse is regularly seen as a definitive action, the one you're working your way toward, the headliner. Yet, actually intercourse isn't the best way to engage in sexual relations. A few people lean toward different sorts of joy, including common masturbation, manual stimulation, and oral sex. A few ladies can't climax from intercourse. A few people can't engage in sexual relations. Ladies with high-hazard pregnancies, those who've quite recently conceived an offspring, and those with certain ailments will be unable to have sex, similarly as men with erectile brokenness or prostate issues may not. Yet, that doesn't mean you can't have intercourse! Toys offer couples the chance to consider some fresh possibilities.

Examination has demonstrated that most of ladies need clitoral stimulation to climax. For certain ladies, a hand or a tongue basically isn't sufficient. They need a ground-breaking, engaged, steady sort of stimulation that people can't generally give. That is the reason vibrators exist! Vibrators convey a specific sort of stimulation that is unequaled. A few ladies locate that oral sex and manual stimulation feel superb, turn them on, and get them to the edge, yet can't convey them into delight. Vibrators can get you to the end goal. For long haul couples, toys can be that sparkle you need to reignite your sexual relationship. Here and there, when you bring something new and new to your sexual coexistence, it encourages you reconnect with your partner. Basically looking for another play item can be an immense turn-on for some couples. As you peruse the racks at a store, you can murmur sexy things to each other, uncover what you like about a specific toy, and bother each other with the potential outcomes. Whenever you've made your buy, there's bounty more enjoyable to come. Every Christmas, a man I know arranges an extraordinary new toy for his better half and incorporates a transcribed card with it; it has become a convention for them. He loves to sort out the ideal one to purchase, while she delights in the expectation of what's sitting tight for her under the tree. They've had an energizing, satisfying sexual coexistence for over fifteen years together.

Deliverer Shapes, swings, and slings can help change the point of entrance or uphold and orchestrate your bodies in manners you never thought conceivable, hence rousing new positions. Things, for example, blindfolds, rub oil candles, and G-spot toys may bring new exercises into your suggestive collection. Toys can likewise make way for dream pretending; now and then everything necessary is a break of the oar to keep mischievous young ladies or young men in line! Eventually, there's an explanation vibrators, dildos, and attachments are called sex toys: They're loads of fun!

Ten Reasons to Add Sex Toys to Your Sex Life

1. Investigate something new: It's anything but difficult to get exhausted or self-satisfied in a drawn out sexual relationship. Kick things up an indent with a sex toy.

2. Go from great to extraordinary: Already having hot sex? Set innovation and development to work for you, and make it much more smoking.

3. Have a fast in and out: Sometimes, you simply need to get off and get off brisk. Why not take an easy route to that delivery and unwinding?

4. Sharing time: Take turns stroking off for one another, each with a most loved toy. You'll will observe one another, flaunt for your partner,

and possibly get familiar with some things about your darling from the exhibition.

5.   Stay up the entire evening: Let's say your penis is accomplished for the night, however you two aren't. Get a toy, and you're all set for the same number of more adjusts as you need.

6.   Bring her over the edge: Some ladies need incredible, relentless clitoral stimulation to come, and a vibrator is the lone thing that will assist them with getting.

7.   Accomplish synchronicity: Want to encounter joy in quite a few spots at a similar specific time? Synchronous sensations (and orgasms) are conceivable!

8.   Go for additional: Whether you need to figure out how to become multiorgasmic or it comes, indeed, normally to you, toys help rouse various orgasms for him and her.

9.   Twofold delight: Is your partner longing for double the fun however you would prefer not to welcome a neighbor over to assist? You can be the two places without a moment's delay with a dildo or vibrator.

10.   Make your own experience: If the room is your stage, consider sex toys the props in your sensual show; be imaginative, have a good time, and grasp your perky side!

CONCLUSION

Maybe the best piece of tantric sex is that it benefits everybody. "Tantra can help men experiencing untimely discharge because it hinders the cycle of sex and eliminates the strain to perform," says Tammy Nelson, Ph.D. authorized psychotherapist, relationship master, and creator of Getting the Sex You Want. "For ladies, figuring out how to unwind and be at the time can help with orgasmic work just as building want." It can likewise help your relationship outside the room by improving close correspondence.

While climaxes aren't the objective, per state, "tantric climaxes" are often alluded to as supernatural encounters, says Sally Valentine, Ph.D., a certified sex specialist in Boca Raton, Florida.

Sign me up, isn't that so? Be that as it may, how the hell do you take the plunge? To begin with, talk it over with your accomplice.

Give them the deets on what it is and why you need to attempt it (you know: further closeness, energy, additionally fulfilling sex, or for no particular reason). When your boo offers the go-ahead, begin joining the specialty of tantra into your sex routine with these straightforward advances.

Sentimental Dinner in Room

Get into the temperament is by joining ceremonies into sex. That can be anything, for example, setting up your space as an asylum with candles, pads, and delicate music.

What's most significant is that you cause sex to feel, well, uncommon. "You need a feeling that sex is something significant and particular from regular day to day existence," state Johnson and Michaels.

Visually Connect

Eye to eye connection will help both of you feel nearer during sex. Zero in on one another. Generally, this is by investigating their left eye, yet you can investigate both if that is more agreeable to you.

Give Each Other Back Rubs

Give each other small scale sexual back rubs. David Yarian, Ph.D., an authorized clinician, and certified sex specialist, suggests exchanging between who gives and gets joy.

For example, you may request that your accomplice give you a foot rub for two minutes, and afterward, you would do whatever your accomplice says they need for two minutes.

During your turn, give your accomplice input (for instance, "to one side," "somewhat more weight would be extraordinary," and so on) Then, when it's your accomplice's turn, urge them to do likewise. "This is a method of rehearsing a component of adoration making deliberately as an approach to learn—figure out how to be the most ideal sweetheart for our accomplice," says Yarian. What's more, the other way around, obviously.

Focus on the Development of Your Body

"Consider what it seems like to move bodies together," says Yarian. Furthermore, make an effort not to pass judgment on anything you notice or contrast it with different encounters you've had—simply center around what you're feeling at the time (instead of, state, considering the climax you're trusting you'll have in almost no time). "This is a method of placing the cerebrum in impartial and relinquishing the reasoning," says Yarian. It's likewise an incredible method to guarantee you don't pass up all the spine-shivering joy that occurs before you get to the end goal.

Postpone Climax

"Deferring climax often intensifies the experience," said Johnson and Michaels. "Staying in a high condition of excitement can likewise assist individuals with encountering vigorous climaxes, or climaxes without discharging," they add.

Deferring a climax implies you carry yourself to the bring of having one, just to chill out and postpone it. Called edging, it's ideal to try it out while stroking off to understand the method. Work on getting yourself up to the point of climax, then halting, and firing up once more. Then, when you're with your accomplice, you can alternate getting each other up toward the peak, sliding down, and afterward returning up again toward climax prior to giving up to the firecrackers finale.

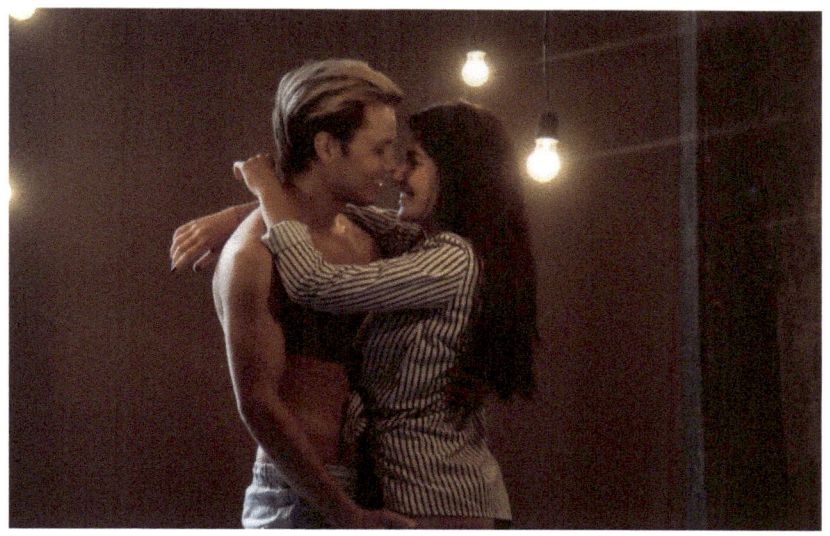